The Rants and Raves of a Hypothyroid Patient

Wishes, Concerns and Lessons-Learned

By: James M. Lowrance © 2010

TABLE OF CONTENTS:

The Rants and Raves of a Hypothyroid Patient

INTRODUCTION:

As a Thyroid Patient Advocate, I contribute to the best of my ability; in inspiring my fellow patients to learn more about their disease and to become better advocates for their own medical care. It has been an observed fact, documented by medical advocacy and research groups, that those patients who practice self-advocacy, experience better treatment outcomes and learn how to better partner with their doctors in their ongoing care.

As a hypothyroid patient myself, I have experienced many of the same struggles my fellow patients go through. This includes symptom struggles that can flare at times despite being well-treated for my hypothyroidism and having disappointing experiences with less-specialized doctors, before finding one that provided me adequate and optimal treatment.

In the chapters of this book, I share some of the more helpful knowledge I gained as a newly diagnosed thyroid patient, beginning in year-2003, to the present.

I also express a few opinions and take a look at some of the controversies that have continued, between medical professionals and patient advocates, in regard to symptoms, diagnosis and treatments for hypothyroidism. Along the way, you'll find that I added a few "rants and raves" in regard to these issues but hopefully, nothing that might be perceived as disrespectful or offensive to either side of the debates.

It is my hope that the readers of this book will find inspiration, encouragement and knowledge, in helping them to become self-advocates and possibly even to join myself and others in the growing number of Thyroid Patient Advocates who help to inspire and encourage others being treated for hypothyroidism.

CHAPTER ONE

Those Crazy Thyroid Antibodies

(When the Immune System Goes Haywire!)

A major cause of thyroid diseases in industrialized countries is "thyroid autoimmunity", meaning cells are being specifically created by the immune system to attack the thyroid gland. This event of mistaken identity in which this major hormone-producing endocrine gland is recognized as an enemy, results in types of thyroiditis, goiters and thyroid hormone imbalances.

As with other autoimmune diseases, the thyroid types also involve antibodies from the immune system that attack the gland as if it is an enemy in the body that needs destroyed. Medical research groups have studied autoimmunity, meaning the process by which these antibodies attack natural areas of the body and they still cannot pin down any definitive answers as to why these diseases occur. It is as though the immune system goes a bit crazy and there is misrecognition of body tissues as invaders that must be eradicated.

The Rants and Raves of a Hypothyroid Patient

It is an amazing thing to begin with, to realize that antibodies can be created by the immune system, to attack specific illness-causing cells that enter the body, such as allergens, bacteria and viruses. If forexample a flu virus is breathed in through the nose and begins to replicate, increasing to large enough numbers in the body to cause influenza symptoms, the immune system will design an antibody to specifically attack that virus. As it does so, it touches nothing else in the body although it does work in cooperation with white blood cells that also help the body to fight-off and recover-from illnesses and infections.

In the case of thyroid autoimmunity, cells of the thyroid gland, usually protein-enzymes that are in the gland that result in the manufacture and distribution of thyroid hormones (i.e. peroxidase and thyroglobulin), are recognized and targeted by the immune system. Antibodies are specially designed to stop the hormone producing process by the attempted eradication of these essential proteins. As this occurs, the thyroid gland becomes damaged and inflamed, resulting in a condition called "autoimmune thyroiditis".

In most cases, the resulting disease is called "Hashimoto's thyroiditis", which is the name of the Japanese medical doctor, who first officially documented cases of the disease in patients he was treating.

Once Dr. Hashimoto's research was confirmed the disease was named in approximately the year 1912. Before this, people who had types of thyroiditis causing inflammation and swelling in the gland were simply termed as having "goiters". While a goiter is still medically recognized today, doctors can now diagnose the diseases that cause them, such as Hashimoto's which results in hypothyroidism (under-active gland) and Graves' disease which results in hyperthyroidism (overactive gland). In countries poor in iodine-rich diets, especially those who do not have access to iodized salt for table-use and cooking, iodine deficiency is a major cause of goiters.

In the industrialized countries of the world, most cases of thyroid disease are caused by those "crazy thyroid antibodies".

CHAPTER TWO:

What it Feels like to be Hypothyroid

(Sunk in a Pit or Run Over by a Truck)

Hypothyroid symptoms can be mild, moderate or severe and the rate at which they manifest can vary among patients. Many people with developing hypothyroidism believe they are simply experiencing aging, stress or lack of rest. The fatigue and depression can be severe however and treatment must be administered.

Symptoms of hypothyroidism – an under-active thyroid gland, manifest differently for each person who experiences it. This condition which results from a state of low thyroid hormone levels causes a person's metabolism to run abnormally slow. Some people notice a slow, worsening onset of their symptoms, while others seem to experience them more suddenly. As a treated hypothyroid patient, I can attest to a slow onset of my initial symptoms but at a certain point, these worsened suddenly.

Like many people with under-active thyroids, I originally believed my symptoms were caused by stress, working too hard and not getting enough sleep.

Hypothyroid symptoms can include those that follow.

- Fatigue tiredness and malaise
- Dry skin and hair
- Weight gain
- Mood changes, especially depression
- Slowed digestion with constipation

The thing that prompted a doctor visit for me was a worsening of emotional symptoms, that in my case I experienced as a mix of both depression and anxiety, with some panic attacks, especially at night while trying to sleep (nocturnal). I began to realize my symptoms were more than just a result of being stress-out and tired and I made doctor visits to have blood testing ordered, which identified my hypothyroidism, caused by autoimmune thyroiditis.

You could say that some people, who develop hypothyroid conditions, basically feel like they've been run over by a truck, while others feel like they slowly sank into a pit of tiredness and depression. Either way, once symptoms become full blown or in medical terms, what they call "overt hypothyroidism", the only thing that will relieve symptoms is getting the low thyroid hormone levels corrected. This is done by taking a prescribed dose of replacement thyroid hormone which is determined by a treating doctor based on the severity of the low hormone levels and the patient's body-size.

Once the patient's body adjusts to the daily dose of hormone which takes about eight weeks - symptoms will begin to improve. Some patients need their dose levels adjusted a time or two before significant symptom-relief is experienced and the treating doctor will know if adjustments need to be made, by monitoring the treatment with repeat blood tests at regular intervals of about 2 to 3 times yearly.

Retests are however ordered more frequently during the first months of treatment, which is usually the phase of treatment requiring more dosage adjustments.

Treatment for hypothyroidism will restore energy, digestion, better weight control and improved mood in patients who are treated.

CHAPTER THREE

Finding a Good Thyroid Doctor

(Physicians who Diagnose & Treat Hypothyroidism)

When I finally broke down with some prompting by my wife, to make a doctor appointment to have my symptoms of chronic fatigue and my mood problems of depression and anxiety investigated, I visited a fill-in MD. My regular MD was out of town preparing to start a practice in a third world country as a missionary doctor and he was in-between seeing patients at his U.S. office. My appointment just happened to be at one of those times he was out of the country.

The doctor who was attending his appointments listened to me describe my symptoms which only took a minute or two and she immediately picked up a prescription pad off of a counter in the examination room and wrote me out three prescriptions. One was for an antidepressant, the other was an anti-anxiety medication and the third was a beta-blocker drug to reduce the effects of adrenaline in my body.

The doctor felt these would help with my anxiety symptoms. My blood pressure, taken by the nurse before the doctor came in, was normal but no other physical tests were done, such as checking my reflexes or listening to my heart.

The doctor informed me that my symptoms indicated "Generalized Anxiety Disorder" and was the reason for the prescribing of the three medications. I asked if possibly some testing could be ordered for me and the doctor reacted a bit offended at my suggestion and replied by saying I could get an MRI of my brain done. Not realizing this was an answer spoken out of disgust that I, as a patient suggested that I needed more thorough medical evaluation; I asked what the cost would be as a non-insured, self-pay patient. She responded by informing me that it would cost about $2,000.00. I instead took the prescriptions to my pharmacy and had them filled.

Once arriving at home, I battled in my mind in regard to starting these medications. I was convinced that my symptoms indicated a physical, medical problem, rather than an emotional-only disorder.

I made the decision to hold off on taking the prescribed drugs until after I could have blood testing ordered. I called a doctor's office who agreed to have the blood tests ran and to have the hospital lab send results to my regular doctor, once he was back in his office to review them. My thyroid panel had two abnormal results on it, indicating hypothyroidism and my doctor noted this in his review letter, once reviewing my results.

I relate this story, to demonstrate the importance in seeing a qualified doctor when experiencing symptoms of the type I was seeking evaluation for. While this is not a fact appreciated by some in the medical field when it is pointed out, some doctors are very basic general practitioners. They can treat colds, flu, indigestion, headaches and other basic problems but when it comes to endocrine disorders (problems in glands that produce hormones, including thyroid) they are sometimes lacking the qualification to diagnose and treat them.

It is important to see an endocrinologist in cases when a thyroid or other endocrine disease is suspected.

A thyroid specializing doctor is the best choice when hypothyroid (underactive) or hyperthyroid (overactive) disorders are a strong probability. In many cases, once proper diagnosis and treatment is lined-out, a regular MD or GP can take over follow-up treatments from there.

CHAPTER FOUR

Thyroid Hormone Brand Controversies

(Which Hypothyroid Therapy is Best?)

I am personally treated with Armour Thyroid™ but my personal belief is that symptom relief and optimized blood levels are the true tests of whether a particular brand of thyroid hormone is working for a patient.

After my diagnosis of hypothyroidism and following my prescribed treatment for it, I began to search and research online regarding the different types of treatments. I found that there were not only patients and medical people who disagreed over which brand or type of thyroid hormone was best but there were actual debates going on in regard to the subject, sometimes very heated ones. I found that there were very firm advocates for synthetic T4 brands of prescribed thyroid hormone, the major brand being "Synthroid™" and there were very firm advocates for natural brands of combination T3 and T4 prescribed hormone, the major brand being "Armour Thyroid™".

The advocates for synthetic T4 treatment were pointing out that this type hormone is more stable once each daily dose is administered and that it has a longer half-life (stays in the body longer) than brands that also contain T3 in them. Since there are also brands of combination T4 and T3, such as "Thyrolar™", this opinion would like apply to that brand as well. Also added into the defense of synthetic T4 was the accusation that natural brands of thyroid hormone may be unreliable as far as pill-to-pill consistency goes. In other words, one pill in a bottle of same dose-size pills might contain more or less hormone than the next pill in the bottle.

The advocates for natural T4 and T3 combination treatment were pointing out that synthetic T4 did not restore bodily metabolism as well as animal-derived hormones do in the natural brands. This they were stating was due to the fact that animal thyroid hormones are bio-identical to that found in humans and that thyroid hormones extracted from animals (usually pigs – porcine source), contain others that the human body needs such as T1, T5, T6 and T7 and calcitonin, which is a hormone involved in calcium and phosphorus metabolism in the body.

What I eventually found however was that some hypothyroid patients cannot take one or the other type/brand due to allergic reactions or sensitivities to them. Each type has types of additives in them that are necessary to process them into tablets and dyes the color them for easy identification of dosage differences and these can be allergens to some people. There are in fact some people who are allergic to pork products of any kind. Some patients also have kosher religious observances and cannot consume porcine-derived products.

Blood testing can show exactly where the levels of T4 and T3 hormones are in correcting bodily metabolism. If symptoms are not improving on a particular brand or blood tests show an ongoing imbalance between the T4 and T3, a patient can be switched to a trial of a different brand and their doctor should be willing to do so. Some research studies have shown that T3 is effective in treating depression when included in hormone therapy for hypothyroid patients. Synthetic brands of T3 are also available and can be added to T4 treatments, in addition to already being available, combined in single tablets. Other patients feel jittery and nervous or have anxiety and panic symptoms due to sensitivity to oral T3 dosing.

All of these facts should be considerations between both doctor and patient, when a brand of thyroid hormone is being considered as treatment for an underactive thyroid gland.

Patients are individuals and should be treated as such when best results are being sought for correcting hypothyroidism.

CHAPTER FIVE

The TSH Blood Test Debate

(Thyroid Stimulating Hormone Controversies)

Thyroid Stimulating Hormone (TSH) is the pituitary gland hormone, sent from the brain to the thyroid gland, to stimulate its production of other hormones that regulate metabolism in the body. Debate has been ongoing as to what level the TSH needs to be, to optimally relieve symptoms in hypothyroid patients.

There has been ongoing debate in regard to what level the TSH level needs to be in treated hypothyroid patients. When a person's thyroid gland becomes underactive, the TSH begins to rise to abnormally high levels, which can be detected by blood testing. When treatment is administered to bring thyroid hormone levels back up to normal via a prescribed dose of T4 and/or T3 thyroid hormone medication, this will suppress the TSH back down into normal values.

So where has the controversy come in, regarding the TSH level in treated hypothyroid patients?

The Rants and Raves of a Hypothyroid Patient

The debate has been in regard to just how low the TSH needs to be, for patients to see significant and best symptom relief (optimal). The range of TSH at blood testing labs if roughly between "0.4 to 4.0mIU/L". If a patient's hypothyroidism has caused their TSH to elevate to 10.0 for example, an administered daily dose of thyroid hormone replacement will lower the level back down into the normal values range. The debate has been in regard to whether a lowest-normal TSH, is a better-optimized treatment level than is a mid-range TSH or high-normal reading, as determined by follow up blood retests, to monitor the treatment.

Using the example lab range mentioned above, of "0.4 to 4.0", the question would be - Will a patient on hormone therapy feel better and regain a more improved state of health with a TSH at 2.0 (mid-range), 1.0 (low-normal) or 0.4 (lowest-normal)? One of the problems that can arise are patients who are under-treated at high-normal TSH levels such as 4.0 and they retain some of their hypothyroid symptoms, such as difficulty losing weight and fatigue.

This is especially a realistic possibility with the fact that the ACE (American College of Endocrinologists) recommended in year-2002, that the highest-normal value at blood testing labs, should not be above "3.0". This they proposed is due to the fact that even readings at that level can indicate mild hypothyroidism.

Another problem that can arise is over-treatment of patients on thyroid hormone doses, by suppressing their TSH level down to readings below "0.4", which can induce hyperthyroid symptoms such as nervousness, rapid heart rate and sweating. This is also referred-to as throtoxicity and can lead to eventual osteoporosis (bone loss) and heart arrhythmias (irregular heart beat).

These are the reasons that many thyroid doctors use a targeted goal for TSH in treating hypothyroid patients that is somewhere between lowest-normal and mid-range. This would be a reading of about "1.0", which is usually a safe level that doesn't present the risk for either under-treatment or over-treatment.

This demonstrates the importance in finding a qualified thyroid doctor who understands the importance of proper TSH suppression in the treatment of hypothyroidism. Better doctors also understand the importance of testing the T4 and T3 thyroid hormone levels, to see how they correlate with the TSH with hormone dose administration, for at least the first 2 or 3 blood retests in newly treated hypothyroid patients.

CHAPTER SIX

Anxiety Symptoms with Autoimmune Hypothyroidism

(Anxious and Nervous Hypothyroid Patients)

While this is not an aspect you often see covered on general medical sources that provide information on hypothyroidism, anxiety symptoms do occur with underactive thyroid glands and is not exclusive to hyperthyroid conditions (overactive).

Medical research articles have stated in numerous studies of hypothyroid patients, that they do experience chronic anxiety symptoms and panic attacks with states of low thyroid hormone. This is especially true when the cause of the hypothyroidism is "thyroid autoimmunity", meaning a gland that becomes diseased, due to an attack perpetrated on it by the immune system. The auto-antibodies that are created by the immune system mistakenly attack the gland relentlessly, until it can no longer function in regulating bodily metabolism.

The body produces less energy from things consumed, including food and oxygen and all bodily functions are slowed-down. This cause of hypothyroidism is the most common in industrialized countries, including the US and the UK. It is most often referred-to as "Hashimoto's thyroiditis".

You would think that a slowed metabolism would cause depression rather than anxiety but many patients report anxiety as a symptom of hypothyroidism, even when it is at a sub-clinical level (mild - not full blown). Medical research studies have observed anxiety symptoms in mild cases of underactive thyroid glands and their conclusions can be found on the websites of reputable medical groups, including the U.S. National Institutes of Health (PubMed). The more basic information sites should pick up on this research and include these facts on their general information resources.

Why would thyroid autoimmunity that leads to progressive hypothyroidism cause anxiety symptoms in some patients?

A major reason is a condition referred-to as "Hashitoxicosis", a condition that causes a temporary phase of hyperthyroidism, due to the presence of an antibody called "Thyroid Stimulating Immunoglobulin" (TSI). Usually Hashimoto's autoimmune thyroiditis, results from two major protein-enzyme destroying antibodies called the "anti-thyroidperoxidase" (TPO) and the "anti-thyroglobulin" (TG) but some patients will also develop the TSI antibodies that are typically found more commonly in patients with autoimmune hyperthyroidism (Graves' disease). For a temporary period of time, the TSI will cause a phase of Hashitoxicosis, before permanent, progressive hypothyroidism takes over.

Another aspect that might be involved in causing anxiety symptoms in hypothyroid patients is a reaction by the adrenal glands to low thyroid hormone in the body. Just as adrenaline increases with episodes of hypoglycemia (low blood glucose) in people with diabetes and pre-diabetic conditions, it can potentially do so with other conditions of low hormone, including thyroid and sex-related ones.

More public education, including that which is available to doctors, should inform of this possibility that anxiety symptoms can be a manifestation of autoimmune hypothyroidism and is not restricted to cases of hyperthyroidism.

CHAPTER SEVEN

Unrealistic Expectations from Hypothyroid Therapy

(Imperfections of Thyroid Hormone Replacement)

When I discovered I had hypothyroidism, the autoimmune type to-boot (Hashimoto's thyroiditis), I began searching the websites of thyroid hormone manufacturers and to study other sources regarding thyroid hormone replacement therapy. After all, I was going to have to take this treatment for the rest of my life and I wanted to know what it was all about.

Most sources I searched regarding prescribed thyroid hormone replacement, made hypothyroid therapy sound almost like some type of miracle cure for a slowed-down metabolism, which is what hypothyroidism is. They made statements to the effect that once a person with an underactive thyroid gland begins taking prescribed hormone, to replace that which is lacking by the person's diseased thyroid gland; they would feel like their old-self in no-time!

The Rants and Raves of a Hypothyroid Patient

Most stated that within 6 to 8 weeks, bodily metabolism would be returned to normal and the symptoms of depression, weight gain, dry skin, constipation and fatigue (the real biggie), would all go back to normal.

Needless to say, I was literally excited to begin my own thyroid hormone therapy, with great expectations of feeling like a new man, within a couple of months! When I experienced less-than adequate symptom relief after starting my treatment, I felt terribly let-down, by less than expected results. I in-fact needed several dose adjustments over a period of about two years, before my restored thyroid hormones reached adequate and optimal levels. Even at this level however, it still takes more effort for me to keep extra weight off and I continue to experience periods of fatigue that I believe to be thyroid-related. I do also have other related health problems, including peripheral neuropathies from long-term vitamin deficiencies that have since been corrected but I have learned over time to distinguish thyroid symptoms from those of my other health issues.

Why in some cases, does thyroid hormone therapy fail to relieve symptoms as adequately as desired, in some hypothyroid patients? There may be a number of factors but in my opinion, the autoimmune aspect of the disease is a factor in symptoms as well and thyroid hormone replacement does not cure or reverse thyroid autoimmunity. The antibodies from the immune system that attack the thyroid gland cause an inflammatory response and sometimes swelling in the gland (goiter). Even mild inflammation in the body can feel like a low-grade fever, with mild achiness and fatigue experienced intermittently as a result of it (thyroiditis flares).

I also believe that it's a strong possibility that an administered dose of thyroid hormone, coming into the body from the outside, is somewhat less-effective than are thyroid hormones that naturally occur in the body. Regardless, we are thankful to medical science for hypothyroid treatment, via replacement thyroid hormone that is available in natural (animal derived) and synthetic (lab developed) types, that our doctors can prescribe to keep us healthier.

Without treatment, hypothyroidism is progressive and eventually life-threatening and though my health is not at the level it was before my thyroid disease onset, I for one am grateful for my treatment.

CHAPTER EIGHT

The Pituitary and Thyroid Gland Balancing Act

(Things that can Change Hormone Levels in the Body)

The pituitary gland is the master thermostat control in the brain. It varies in how much "thyroid stimulating hormone" (TSH) it sends to the thyroid gland, according to even the smallest changes in the body, including those caused by things in the diet and exercise levels. TSH is the hormone that tells the thyroid how much of its own hormone to send-out for regulating bodily metabolism in response to these type things.

Thyroid hormone coming into the body from an outside source, such as a prescribed dose can change the pituitary response as well (i.e. thyroid hormone replacement therapy for treatment of hypothyroidism). This is why it's important to take the dose consistently at same time each day, being careful not to take calcium or iron too close to thyroid dosing because these can hinder its absorption in the body.

They should be taken (even if they're just in a multi-vitamin), at least six hours apart from the dose.

I feel, that if a dose of replacement hormone doesn't adjust well in the body for whatever reason, the pituitary compensates by releasing more TSH. Once it does this to increase the thyroid glands production of T4 and T3 (the thyroid hormones), any thyroid gland tissue still intact and not too-diseased to produce hormone, will increase these levels. By the time the levels go up a bit and a next oral dose is taken, these clash a bit and a patient can feel a bit hyperthyroid for a few hours or even days. That's how sensitive this endocrine gland loop is!

Also things such as "goitrogen foods" can affect the loop a bit as well. These are foods that have a natural lowering effect on thyroid hormone in the body so small portions are recommended, rather than consuming large amounts of them. Thoroughly cooking them helps as well (i.e. the cruciferous vegetable types), to reduce their thyroid hormone lowering effects.

The list of "goitrogen foods" is pretty big and you may be disappointed to find out what some of these are, which include the following.

- Broccoli
- Brussel sprouts
- Cabbage
- Cauliflower
- Kale
- Kohlrabi
- Mustard
- Rutabaga
- Turnips
- Millet
- Peaches
- Peanuts
- Radishes
- Soybean products
- Spinach
- Strawberries

The effects these foods can have on lowering thyroid hormone levels can however be avoided by only consuming small amounts of them that are well-cooked (if cooking applies).

I even feel increasing one's exercise level suddenly, rather than gradually over days or weeks can also affect the pituitary-thyroid loop and cause an orally-dosed hypothyroid patient to experience hypothyroid symptoms that may waver back toward hyperthyroid ones, as the pituitary gland tries to compensate. This can occur before they level-out to more of an even keel (euthroid state).

It's all really interesting and as one continues to search this subject, they will find even more of these type facts. It also demonstrates that hypothyroid treatment via hormone replacement therapy is not near as simple as some doctors and medical sources would lead you to believe! Lifestyle practices can indeed have an effect on supplemented thyroid hormones in the body.

CHAPTER NINE

Vitamin Deficiency Neuropathies in Thyroid Patients

(Peripheral Nerve Damage and Low Nutrients)

I recently corresponded with a fellow thyroid patient who has hypothyroidism from Hashimoto's thyroiditis as I do (thyroid autoimmunity disease) and co-morbid (associated) neurological symptoms. We were discussing the fact that vitamin and other nutritional deficiencies can contribute-to or directly cause peripheral neuropathies and that this occurs more often in thyroid disease patients, than in the general public.

Following below, was my description of being diagnosed with vitamin deficiencies when I was being evaluated by a neurologist for the cause of my neuropathy symptoms:

"My diagnosed deficiencies include vitamin D and I've read medical research linking D-deficiency to Hashimoto's thyroiditis developing in some patients.

The Rants and Raves of a Hypothyroid Patient

I am not surprised that there is research saying the opposite, that over-supplementation of vitamin D can cause it, as you mentioned finding through your online medical information search. My D blood result was at "17" and if I remember correctly, the lab range was "25 to 100" but the lab report mentioned that even a "30" reading is considered "insufficient" (close to deficiency).

My other deficiency - the worst one was vitamin E. My blood lab result on it via a neurologist, who ordered it, was "0.4" (less than a half point!) and the normal range is "3.0 to 16.0". Medical sources all state that E-deficiency causes neurological damage, usually peripheral neuropathies.

My third low vitamin which they placed in the "insufficiency" category (as opposed to deficiency) was my B12 level. My reading on it was "374" in a range of "200 to 1100" but the Quest Diagnostics blood lab, noted on the result sheet that readings between 200 and 400 can cause psycho-neurological symptoms.

My neuromuscular symptoms, which seem to be somewhat better at times but definitely still there, are cramping feelings in them, muscle twitches, pinch type sensations in the arches of my feet, tingling at times and stabbing pains. I can feel the pain in my heels often and sometimes they send a vibrating/buzzing sensation that goes all the way up to my hips (not often).

I also have muscle weakness in my arms and legs and my thumbs feel at times as if I've strained the muscles in them and I've had carpal tunnel (wrists/hands) and tarsal tunnel (ankles/feet) type problems on occasion as well.

I worried intensely for a while, thinking I might have something like ALS (Motor Neuron Disease) but I've had these symptoms on and off for far too long (over 7 years but milder, previously), without seeing any apparent muscle atrophy. A spinal tap (lumbar puncture) my neurologist performed on me, ruled out MS, which in-reality does not manifest like these type symptoms that you and I both describe experiencing.

It was nice to have run across that thread in which you describe symptoms very similar to mine (not for you of course but nice to relate to same scenario in a fellow-patient). I too have fairly high thyroid antibodies, revealed by blood tests but my higher one is usually the TG (anti-thyroglobulin) which has been at "537" and in the upper 300s, etc..., so never really drops to a low number. My TPO only has shown elevations up to about "120" but is still significantly above the <35 lab range (anything above 35 being positive for thyroid autoimmunity).

I asked to be tested for antibodies that might indicate that my vitamin deficiencies are liver bile duct dysfunction (a cause of nutrient malabsorption) but I was negative, plus I do not have the symptoms of biliary cirrhosis (autoimmune bile duct disease). I will say that if you haven't had B12, D, E and maybe even B6 blood tested, you might consider doing so, since these vitamins are low in thyroid patients more often than in the healthy public."

CHAPTER TEN

Review for: "The Thyroid Diet" - by Mary Shomon

(Weight Loss Plans for Treated Hypothyroid Patients)

As a Thyroid Patient Advocate, I am inspired to refer readers of my own books and e-books, to other highly valuable and reputable resources. The review I am adding via this chapter is just such a resource, authored by the world's most well-known Thyroid Patient advocate.

In this wonderfully written book by Mary Shomon, one of the most concerning problem-areas for thyroid patients is addressed in detail, namely the problem with weight gain and difficulty losing weight. This is a common complaint heard from treated thyroid patients who find that it requires a great deal more effort for them to control their weight, than before they experienced the onset of thyroid disease. As a male hypothyroid patient, I too can attest to an ongoing struggle with weight loss/control.

I also see the added importance in addressing this problem with the fact that thyroid patients are at higher risk for other metabolic related diseases, including diabetes. These are the reasons this book is such an important resource for thyroid patients to take advantage of.

The Thyroid Diet Part I:

In Part I of Mary's book, she begins by covering information on the symptoms, diagnosis and treatments for thyroid conditions because a weight problem can arise in people who are unaware that they have thyroid conditions. This part of the book looks at risk factors for thyroid disease, missed cases of thyroid dysfunction due to improper testing to detect it and people who have borderline thyroid conditions that doctors may not be willing to treat. All thyroid conditions are discussed in this section of the book, including hypothyroidism (under-active thyroid), hyperthyroidism (some treatments result in hypothyroidism), goiter, nodules and thyroid cancer and how these are also treated.

She also includes information in this section on challenges that may arise in getting properly diagnosed due to doctors who may not order all the necessary tests. She points out that in addition to TSH, tests for thyroid antibodies (for thyroid autoimmunity) and testing of Reverse T3 and TRH (Thyrotrophin Releasing Hormone) to monitor conversion of T4 into T3 in the body may also be needed. Mary discusses treatment for hypothyroidism and looks at the different types of thyroid hormone replacement therapies that are available and the importance of optimized treatment for best results.

Good nutrition and natural supplements are included subjects in this section, including vitamins, minerals and other natural helps that can be incorporated into treatment for hypothyroidism. It was great to see information included on things you should avoid in your diet, including "goitrogen foods" (listed in the book) which can contribute to goiter and reduced thyroid hormone levels.

The Thyroid Diet Part II:

In Part II of the book, Mary gives wonderful, easy-to-understand but detailed explanation describing the metabolic process of food being converted into energy for the body (metabolism and gluconeogenesis). She includes information on the role of insulin, glucagons, leptin, ghrelin, cortisol and adrenaline (metabolic hormones) in this process and how imbalances developing in these delicately balanced hormones, can lead to problems with weight gain and health disorders, including metabolic syndrome and diabetes.

She goes on to describe what it means to be "metabolically efficient", meaning you strike a proper balance between the proper foods you eat, proper aerobic exercise, proper nutrition and hydration and taking into account menopause, which can highly effect hormonal balance in affected women. Inflammatory response in the body is also discussed and how it can point to hormonal imbalance and affect weight control in the body (an aspect I found highly interesting).

The Thyroid Diet Part III:

Mary further addresses weight loss issues (hindrances) in Part III of the book, giving further attention to blood sugar balance, the effects of allergies (including food intolerances) and toxins on metabolism. I was especially interested in the included information on the adrenal hormone imbalance subject, where she discusses "Adrenal Fatigue" which occurs commonly in thyroid patients.

A common fungus overgrowth problem (yeast infection) is also discussed which is caused by the candida fungus, referred to as "Candidiasis" and can be a result of too much refined sugar in the diet. Mary discusses treatments for this yeast overgrowth that can hinder weight loss, including diet changes and natural supplements that can help including probiotics and anti-fungal drugs required in more severe cases.

Another common health disorder negatively affecting digestion and the body's ability to absorb nutrients is addressed called "Celiac Disease".

This is a chronic disorder caused by an allergy to gluten (wheat, barley, rye and possibly oat products). Mary points out that even without having this disease, people can be gluten intolerant with similar negative results and that if it is suspected, tests to diagnose the problem may be needed so that a gluten-free diet can be started to help in recovery and prevention of the disease-effects. She also points out that parasites (parasitic infections) can have negative effects on metabolism and weight control, as can an imbalance between zinc and copper levels in the body.

Tests that can determine a patient's status in these areas are discussed as are treatments and diet-change options to resolve the problems when found. Mary includes information on prescription drugs that can contribute to weight gain and lists a number of natural supplements that can help with weight loss. Also included is a look at mind-body and spiritual aspects that can contribute to overall balance of health. She also goes into the subject of stress, anxiety and depression (these can also affect metabolism).

She gives an overview in regard to prescription drugs that can be administered for problems in this area, when they are resistant to natural supplements, diet and exercise.

Cognitive Behavioral Therapy (CBT) is included as a subject as well as self-help relaxation techniques, deep breathing, Emotional Freedom Techniques (EFT) and other stress reducers. Finally, Mary gives a great run down in regard to exercise, things that can hinder your ability to get proper exercise and how to overcome those and benefit the best possible from a proper exercise regimen.

The Thyroid Diet Parts IV and V:

In Parts IV and V, Mary helps readers to look at options for developing the best possible diet plan for their individual needs. These sections contain informative graphs breaking down the details of each diet plan and includes a check list that helps you determine the best diet for you as an individual. A Body Mass Index is also included to help you determine your best weight level in setting a realistic goal to achieve your desired weight.

The nice thing about these sections is that you can try different options if one doesn't work the desired results for you.

She also suggests lots of recipes with a breakdown chart for each, showing the amounts of calories, fats, carbohydrates, fiber, sugar and protein they contain. She also points out foods high in protein, those that are low-glycemic (low sugar, starch and fat) and provides a chart that distinguishes between beneficial and non-beneficial fats. Also found are suggestions on how to determine the size portions you eat of the foods you choose, the importance of including proper amounts of fiber, water and positive hope/attitude.

She includes chapters on more specialized diets and procedures that patients may consider when weight loss is especially difficult, including prescription weight loss drugs when needed. She also helps us identify those things we need to avoid in our diets, including alcohol, caffeine, refined sugars and some artificial sweeteners.

It's hard to know where to stop in this review because there is so much great information in this book and I've barely scratched the surface.

The Rants and Raves of a Hypothyroid Patient

I'll simply end in saying it is a great overall resource to help thyroid patients develop an effective weight loss plan and diet for improved health and quality-of-life. With so many suggestions and options included, you're sure to find the right plan for weight loss and weight control in this remarkable book and it is available through major book sellers.

My Personal Struggle with Thyroid-Related Weight Gain

I thought I would add a short response I made to a fellow hypothyroid patient with Hashimoto's thyroiditis (same disease as I have), who wrote me in regard to the struggle treated patients have with attempted weight loss and difficulties with preventing weight-gain. In their correspondence with me, they mentioned that they felt the "thyroid autoimmunity" aspect of Hashimoto's disease, might be a factor in weight gain, rather than abnormal thyroid hormone levels alone. This especially being a possibility they felt, with the fact that treated patients continue to struggle with their weight even after they have been returned to a normal state of metabolism via a prescribed daily thyroid hormone replacement dose.

Following below was my response/reply to this opinion (Note: also added to my reply that follows, is a brief mention of peripheral neuropathies, treated hypothyroid patients sometimes continue to experience – a subject covered previously, in Chapter Nine).

"I had read about the "increased hunger" symptom with hypothyroidism before as you had but not in relation to Hashimoto's - the thyroid autoimmunity part of the disease. I have articles out there in regard to symptoms being caused by the antibodies and not just abnormal thyroid hormone levels but it makes sense that increased hunger can be one of them.

I too gained weight with my thyroid disease and my current doctor, a lady who has seen a lot of hypothyroid patients, said she had heard about the difficulty losing weight from many other patients besides me. The intense hunger thing has happened to me in the past, although not very recent. My main problem in the weight-gain area, is eating too much and too often, regardless of my hunger level, so is likely a comfort, stress-relief type thing in my case.

I do know for a fact that I have more difficulty losing weight than before my hypothyroidism, in fact when I was a lot younger I actually purposefully tried to gain because I was too thin for a number of years.

I'm now significantly overweight but not huge. I'm 6ft and 240lb but I carry it well because I'm a bit lanky and it gains all over me, rather than just in my middle, so people are always surprised when I tell them my weight.

It's amazing that your blood thyroid antibody levels are in the 1,000s! I've heard other patients attest to levels that high and from what I've read, those levels don't place you in danger of anything in-particular but can increase inflammation levels in your body, making you feel like a person does when they have a low-grade fever. It could be however, as you've suggested, that high elevation can contribute to weight gain.

I need to click and read your other email, which I believe had mention of pituitary gland involvement in the title but I did also want to mention a Med-Help forum thread I found.

The thread was titled "POLL/Neuropathy & Thyroid-Please Join", in which a woman with autoimmune hypothyroidism appealed to other hypothyroid patients, wanting them to express if they were having peripheral neuropathy (PN) symptoms. She received 80 replies!

This many replies to a forum-thread are not typical, which means lots of Hashimoto's-hypothyroid patients are experiencing PN symptoms. Some of them say in the posts that doctors need to realize how many of us have this manifestation with our disease because as it is, they think PN is not related to thyroid if your hormone levels have been corrected back to normal (once the euthroid state is achieved). This is yet another proof that thyroid antibodies play a role in the symptoms of hypothyroidism, such as weight gain and neuropathies and not abnormal hormone levels alone"

(End of Reply)

CHAPTER ELEVEN
Thyroid Patient Self-Advocacy is Essential

(Being a Proactive Hypothyroid Patient)

I have autoimmune hypothyroid disease and I was also diagnosed with Chronic Fatigue Syndrome co-morbid (co-occurring) to it. I've had struggles at times getting proper treatment and without trying to sound too derogatory toward doctors, some of them are not as updated on their knowledge and treatments as they should be. Many thyroid patients go through 4 or 5 doctors before finding one that can treat thyroid problems adequately or optimally. For me, it was the 5th one that I ended up keeping because she works with me better than all of the previous ones.

I really believe the best thing for a newly diagnosed patient, is to get set-up with an Endocrinologist or doctor of whatever MD title that specializes in thyroid treatments. Some Endo-doctors do however treat/specialize in diabetes and thyroid disease is less of a specialty for them.

In my opinion a doctor needs to be questioned in regard their area of expertise before a patient makes a final decision in choosing one for treatment.

Because of problems patients have getting doctors who are specialized and who have the compassion to listen to them rather than sloughing them off with mediocre or less care, patients have to be proactive in their treatment or it will most-likely be inadequate. I know this sounds cynical but I've learned this through correspondence with 1,000s of other thyroid patients since the year 2003. This is not to say there aren't terrific doctors out there because there are many but patients have to pay attention to where their treatment is going because there are doctors who under-treat their patients. There's also such a thing as over-treatment but this happens far less often because some doctors would rather keep patients slightly hypothyroid than hyperthyroid.

The ways patients self-advocate and partner with their doctors, are by also self-educating about thyroid hormone replacement treatment.

You find out what the better specialists out there state as being the level a treating doctor needs to place your TSH and thyroid hormone levels at (T4 and T3) with replacement hormone. Patients who feel this is too much trouble may be forfeiting better treatment. Most doctors will listen to patients who have some knowledge about their treatment and who suggest to their doctor where they believe their treatment levels need to be. The doctor of course would want any adjustment in treatment to remain within normal values (normal lab ranges) but would likely be willing to give a patient trials of doses that help better optimize their treatment.

What I've been doing as a Thyroid Patient Advocate, online, is to take the better information out there offered by The American Association of Clinical Endocrinologists, the National Institutes of Health and well known, reputable Endocrinologists/MDs and helping get that info out to fellow patients. It also came from my own struggle with getting proper treatment and with certain symptoms that were difficult to get resolved even with proper/adequate and even optimal treatment.

It also came from the fact that co-morbid conditions often happen with thyroid disease, other things can branch off from it in other words, like CFS, fatty liver, diabetes and other autoimmune and endocrine diseases but patients are often not informed of these risks by their doctors. I wanted to know everything about how this disease might affect me and I did so by years of online search.

Patients have a right to know everything about a disease that affects their lives!

CHAPTER TWELVE

Respectful Thyroid Patient Advocacy

(Representing Fellow Hypothyroid Sufferers)

What is a "Thyroid Patient Advocate"? Well an "advocate" of any kind, is someone who represents another or others, in a specific cause. A "Thyroid Patient Advocate", not only represents thyroid patients but also is a patient their self and so this can give them the same perspective in many ways that other patients have.

Thyroid Patient Advocates also go-to-bat, so to speak for other patients by representing their needs before the medical community when possible. They will also help to provide informative resources of information and support that will help other patients, in regard to their disease and its treatment.

In this chapter, I wanted to express some things in regard to what is called "thyroid patient advocacy", that is out there across the worldwide web (online).

Sometime ago, people began referring to me as a "Thyroid Patient Advocate" because of my having a significant number of articles on thyroid subjects, published on several thyroid websites. Since being recognized in this way, I've wanted to represent thyroid patients in a respectful way because I see some things coming from fellow-advocates, that are concerning to me and these are things that instead of furthering and improving medical help for thyroid patients, can backfire at times, causing thyroid patient advocacy to at-times be viewed in a bad light.

I feel it is important that advocates do their best to keep this from happening because if we instead approach advocacy in a respectful way but also at the same time, state our beliefs and desires for thyroid treatment, firmly, continually and with strong conviction, I feel this will much better further our cause. The constant attacks that some in patient-advocacy feel they need to perpetrate toward people in the medical field, in my opinion does not accomplish this.

Not long ago, one Thyroid Patient Advocate in an e-mail accused me of "kissing up" to the medical community (exact words).

She claimed I was not joining more in the attacks against medical professionals. I pointed out to this person that there will be more recognition for what we have to say, if we are not on the attack but instead, respectfully express our views with strong conviction. After all, everyone in the medical field, relating to thyroid issues are not bad people. There are good, caring, quality medical professionals who are truly out for the patient's interests. This is why, when I see an attack-article directed at an organization such as the AACE (American Association of Clinical Endocrinologists) or some other organization as a whole, it disappoints me. There are good and bad representatives in every field that exists and we cannot generalize everyone into one category.

There are people within any organization worthy of rebuke but the generalizing I just referred-to, is not fair. This would be like saying all Thyroid Patient Advocates are bad or all doctors are bad, all police etc…, and I do not want the general public of thyroid patients to perceive this as a "Thyroid Patient Advocates, against the Medical Community" agenda.

We could come across as whiners and complainers but we will get far more attention if we are viewed as those who respectfully disagree with strong conviction in certain areas regarding thyroid disease treatments.

Advocates also need to not fall apart and fly off the handle, simply because someone in the medical field disagrees with something they may be expressing in their books or articles, especially when they may do the same thing on-occasion in regard to information written by medical professionals. In the past, I left several thyroid forums that degraded into attacks, gossip and tabloid type behaviors and this-too, was a black eye to thyroid advocacy in my opinion. These posts are often permanently indexed on the search engines and will not have a positive effect on patient-advocacy efforts.

Let both sides of an issue be expressed and then let the chips fall where they may (I would suggest) because over time, the right message will be proven correct. We need to continue putting-out the information we feel is important and the medical community will continue to do the same.

Let these two communities decipher between
what they feel is right or wrong and hopefully if
we continue to do this, over time we will see
changes that really do need to happen in regard to
treatments. If we attack and are continually
disrespectful, when offering our information from
patient-perspectives, it will cause nothing but
more resistance to changes that really do need to
happen. The medical community is after all, the
entity with the knowledge and ability to develop
medical treatments. Without them, we patients
would have little hope.

Many of us patients, including myself have
expressed anger regarding treatment we have
received from a particular doctor (sometimes
more than one) that was obviously bad but this is
not quit the same thing. I for example, was over-
dosed by a doctor with my prescribed thyroid
hormone, to the point that my blood levels of the
hormone were more than double the highest
normal range. This placed me at risk for
dangerous heart arrhythmias, hypertension and
osteoporosis. This occurred despite my request for
blood retests to be conducted much sooner due to
my symptoms of over-treatment but my doctor
continually failed to order them.

The Rants and Raves of a Hypothyroid Patient

In cases like these, we are able to point out and educate between good and obviously bad treatment, without too much generalizing, being careful to also point out that good treatment is always available through the right doctor. We can express our disagreements about what we believe to be inadequate treatments, in a firm but respectful way and without too much negative-generalizing of medical doctors.

It is important that we as Thyroid Patient Advocates are persistent and determined because there are better possibilities for improved treatments for thyroid patients, in our future, as a result but let's work together with the medical community as a whole and not against it. There will always be the "bad apples" in every field, possibly even including those in patient-advocacy but there are also those you can find common ground with, in joining together to see improved treatments for thyroid patients.

(END)

www.ingramcontent.com/pod-product-compliance
Lightning Source LLC
Chambersburg PA
CBHW020403290526
45785CB00005B/2425